Bodybuilding Nutrition How To Build Muscle And Burn Fat Fast

Nutrition Manual

by

George Moller

Table of Contents

Chapter 1: Tools We Will Be Using For Progress Tracking

Progress tracking is one vital aspect of pretty much anything in life, as the saying goes If you can't measure it, you can't manage it. We want to be in full control of what we are doing, we don't want to be guessing. In this chapter, we will answer the following two questions:

1. How do I measure my progress?
2. How often should I measure my progress?

To go even further we need to break down the first question into these three:

1. How can I track the food I eat every day?
2. How can I track my weight?
3. How can I track my body fat percentage?

1.1 How To Track Your Food

When it comes to food, we need to track two things, first is the weight of the food we are eating every day and second is its macronutrients (carbohydrates, protein, fats). The second being dependent of the first of course, so we are going to need two tools here:

1. A food scale to track the weight of each food. 2. My Fitness Pal (mobile app) or journal to track the macronutrients of the food we weight.

As I am going to explain in further chapters the number of macronutrients (proteins, carbohydrates and fats) we consume per day plays a huge role in muscle building and fat lose, so keeping track of them becomes a vital task.

For now, what you need to know is that each and every one of the foods we consume has a certain number of macronutrients which varies depending on the weight of this particular food. For example, 100 grams of chicken breast has roughly 31 grams of protein, 0 grams of carbohydrate, 3.6 grams of fat and 165 calories.

The scale helps us to weight our food hence to know how much protein, carbohydrates, fats and calories we are consuming in each meal. Once we weighted a particular food, say we are having 150 grams of breast chicken for lunch, we pull up my fitness pal and search for chicken breast and enter the amount, in this case 150 grams, then the app will give us the macronutrients for that particular food at that particular weight. You don't have to use my fitness pal you could just keep a food journal of what you are eating every day, (bear in mind that you will have to search in google for the macronutrients of the food, just type the name of the food plus the words "nutrition facts" and google will show you the macronutrients).

So yes, you need to incorporate two new habits in your life now, and at first it might seem that it takes forever to weight the food and enter its information in the app or writing it down in a journal but believe me, like with anything in life at first it may seem complicated but as time goes by you will get more and more used to doing this. I remember when I first started, it was not easy but with time I memorized most of the food information that I consume on a daily basis. Just remember that you don't need to be one hundred percent accurate with your numbers, at least at first, a rough approximation is just fine.

You can start by tracking your calories first and not the macronutrients, once you get used to tracking your calories move on to tracking the protein for each meal, then track your carbohydrates and fats. If you try to keep track of calories and macronutrients at first you might get unmotivated and probably giving up on the whole process.

Let's move to question number two.

1.2 How to track your weight

The answer is pretty obvious here, a bathroom scale.

1.3 How to track your body fat percentage

First let's briefly explain what body fat is. Body fat is the amount of fat that carries in our bodies. Simple as that. A body fat test is an attempt to separate every pound of our body into one of two categories: your fat mass and everything else. What isn't fat mass is considered lean body mass which consists of your bones, muscles, hair, water, etc.

For the average person that doesn't have access to a DEXA scan (the most accurate method to calculate your body fat percentage) the following two methods are the most accurate:

1. Skin-fold method
2. Skulpt

Skin-fold method

The skin fold estimation methods are based on a skin fold test, also known as a pinch test, whereby a pinch of skin is precisely measured by calipers at several standardized points on the body to determine the subcutaneous fat layer thickness. This is what calipers look like:

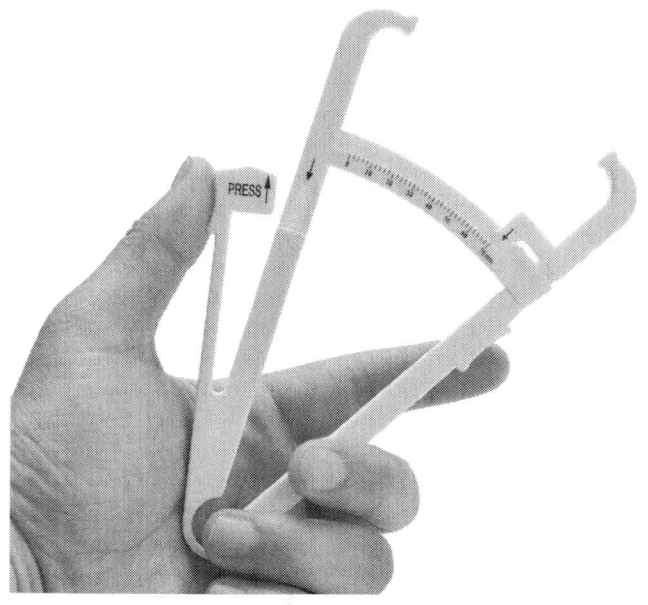

So, once you get a caliper you should measure your abdominal subcutaneous fat by:

1. Placing the calipers about 1 cm to the side of your fingers. Use the pictures below for examples.

2. Pressing on the serrated thumb pad next to the word "press" until the two arrows line up.

3. Noting the measurement on the little scale to the right of the arrows. The hashes are in increments of two. That means one mark lower than 20 is 18.

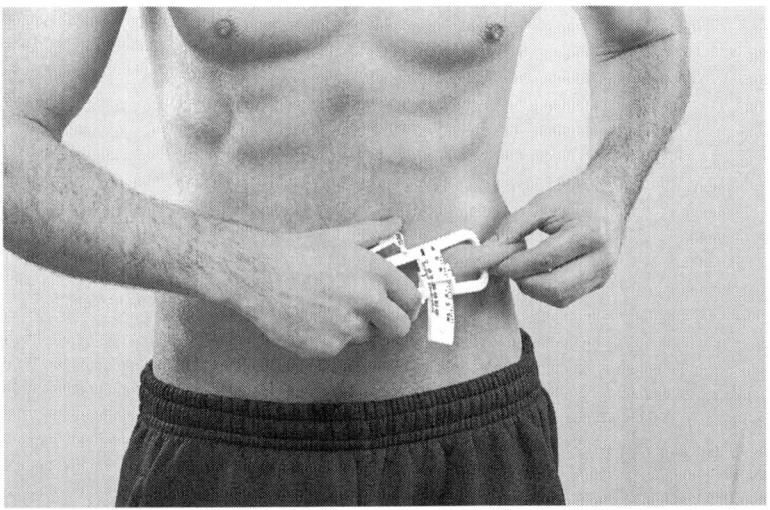

Once you have your measurement you need to check the following table to get an estimated body fat percentage:

Age	Reading in Milliimiters																
	2-3	4-5	6-7	8-9	10-11	12-13	14-15	16-17	18-19	20-21	22-23	24-25	26-27	28-29	30-31	32-33	34-36
18-20	11.3	13.5	15.7	17.7	19.7	21.5	23.2	24.8	26.3	27.7	29.0	30.2	31.3	32.3	33.1	33.9	34.6
21-25	11.9	14.2	16.3	18.4	20.3	22.1	23.8	25.5	27.0	28.4	29.6	30.8	31.9	32.9	33.8	34.5	35.2
26-30	12.5	14.8	16.9	19.0	20.9	22.7	24.5	26.1	27.6	29.0	30.3	31.5	32.5	33.5	34.4	35.2	35.8
31-35	13.2	15.4	17.6	19.6	21.5	23.4	25.1	26.7	28.2	29.6	30.9	32.1	33.2	34.1	35.0	35.8	36.4
36-40	13.8	16.0	18.2	20.2	22.2	24.0	25.7	27.3	28.8	30.2	31.5	32.7	33.8	34.8	35.6	36.4	37.0
41-45	14.4	16.7	18.8	20.8	22.8	24.6	26.3	27.9	29.4	30.8	32.1	33.3	34.4	35.4	36.3	37.0	37.7
46-50	15.0	17.3	19.4	21.5	23.4	25.2	26.9	28.6	30.1	31.5	32.8	34.0	35.0	36.0	36.9	37.6	38.3
51-55	15.6	17.9	20.0	22.1	24.0	25.9	27.6	29.2	30.7	32.1	33.4	34.6	35.6	36.6	37.5	38.3	38.9
56 & UP	16.3	18.5	20.7	22.7	24.6	26.5	28.2	29.8	31.3	32.7	34.0	35.2	36.3	37.2	38.1	38.9	39.5
	LEAN				IDEAL				AVERAGE				ABOVE AVERAGE				

Congratulations! You have an estimated value for your body fat percentage. You can now check in which category do you fall into.

If you don't have a caliper yet, below there is an image where you can have a not very accurate but at least an idea of your body fat percentage:

[6]

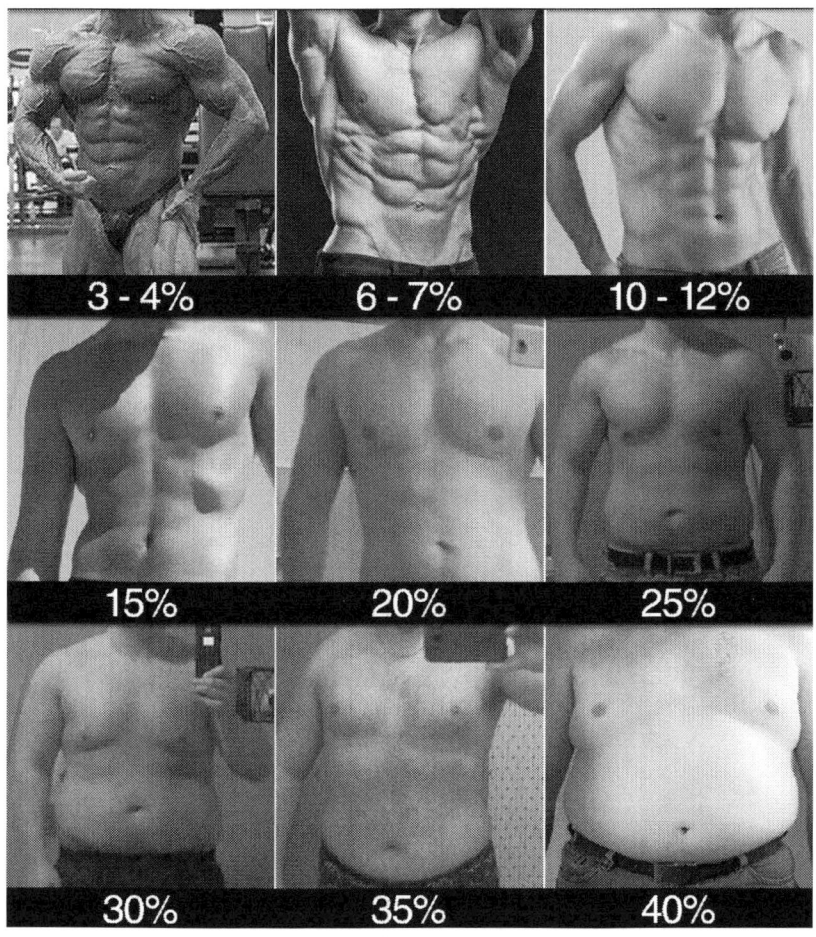

Skulpt

Skupt is a device that can measure your overall body fat percentage and muscle quality, and the fat percentage and muscle quality for each individual muscle as well. It comes with a mobile app which you can sync with the Skupt and keep track of your body fat from your phone. I have it myself and I find it to be really useful.

For more information about the Skulpt please check:

https://www.skulpt.me/

1.4 How Often Should You Keep Track Of Your Progress?

I usually weight myself every day, first thing in the morning before having breakfast but there is no need to do this every day, you can keep track of your weight by weighting yourself once a week, and as long as you see progress (weight gain if your goal is to increase muscle and weight lose if you want lose fat) you'll be just fine. Take into account that the scale is not the best way to measure progress, because weight gain doesn't necessarily mean that you are gaining muscle and weight lose doesn't necessarily mean you are losing fat, you could be gaining fat instead of muscle, and losing muscle instead of fat. That's why it is important to also measure your body fat percentage along with your weight.

In every so call bulking phase[1], you will gain muscle and a little bit of fat along with it, that's completely natural, we just need to make sure the fat gain is minimal compared to the muscle gain. The same goes with fat, in every so call cutting phase[2], you will lose a little bit of muscle along with the fat, but then again we just need to make sure that the muscle loss is minimal. We do this with proper nutrition plans, which I am going to cover in further chapters.

So, how do you make sure you are gaining muscle or losing fat? Weight yourself once a week, and re measure your body fat percentage.

For example, if our goal is to gain muscle, and on week one you weight 154 pounds (70kg) at 12% body fat, then after one week let's say you weight 155 pounds (70.45kg) at 12.2% body fat, your lean muscle mass at the beginning was 135.52 pounds (61.6 kg) [154 - (154 * 0.12)] and at the end of week one is 136.09 pounds (61.85kg) [155 - (155 * 0.122)]. From this you can know for sure that you gain 136.09 - 135.52 = 0.57 pounds of lean muscle mass, but also gain 18.91 (amount of body fat at the end of week one) - 18.48 (amount of body fat at the beginning) = 0.43 pounds of body fat.

To sum up:

1. The smart way to keep track of your progress is to weight yourself and re measure your body fat percentage at least once a week before breakfast.

2. The fact that you are gaining weight every week doesn't necessarily mean that all of that new weight is lean muscle mass.

3. The fact that you are losing weight every week doesn't necessarily mean that all of that weight loss comes from fat.

[1]. Bulking: refers to the process of building lean muscle mass.
[2]. Cutting: refers to the process of dropping body fat.

Chapter 2: Training or Nutrition: Which one is more important?

There are different schools of thought about this, some will say that building muscle or losing weight is 80% nutrition and 20% training, others will say it's a 50% 50% ratio. What I have never heard of is someone giving more importance to training than nutrition. There's a saying among strength coaches and personal trainers *"You can't out-train a lousy diet!"*.

When I first started lifting (10 years ago) I pretty much focused all of my attention to my workout and training, neglecting my nutrition. After three years of little to no gains whatsoever, I decided to educate myself about nutrition, about how to eat to gain muscle and be healthy. That was a huge game changer for me, I was able to put on more muscle in one year of training than I did in the previous three.

I found out that if you get your nutrition right but your workout is not perfect, you can still make amazing gains but it doesn't work the other way around, at least it didn't for me.

So, my advice is, if you're a beginner and you don't possess nutritional knowledge, then mastering nutrition is far more important than training and should become your number one priority. I say this because improving a poor diet can create rapid, quantum leaps in fat loss and muscle building progress.

[11]

No matter how hard you train or what type of training routine you're on, it's all in vain if you don't provide yourself with the right nutritional support. In beginners (or in advanced trainees who are still eating poorly), these changes in diet are more likely to result in great improvements than a change in training.

Remember that what you do when you workout is to break down muscle tissue, you are not actually making your muscles bigger. Muscle recovery occurs after your workout and it depends entirely on how on point are your nutrition and rest.

If you are an intermediate or advanced trainee who has the nutrition in place, changes in your training become much more important, relatively speaking. Your training must become downright scientific.

So, to answer the question, while nutrition is **always** critically important, it's more important to emphasize for the beginner (or the person whose diet is still not in place), while training is more important for the advanced person.

Once you've mastered nutrition, then it's all about keeping that nutrition consistent and progressively increasing the efficiency and intensity of your workouts.

It's not that nutrition ever ceases to be important, the point is, further improvements in nutrition won't have as much impact once you already have all the fundamentals in place.

Chapter 3: Fundamentals

3.1 The 4 Worst Mistakes To Avoid If You Want To Gain Muscle

3.1.1 Mistake 1: Eat Big To Get Big

I heard a lot of pro bodybuilders giving this advice to people. I don't know if you are aware but 99 % of IFBB pro bodybuilders and athletes are steroid users, so they can afford to eat big to get big, but the rules that apply to them don't apply to natural bodybuilders, not at all. They can get away with eating tons of calories per day because their bodies burn much more calories than the natural lifter. If you were to follow this so call "advice" you would end up putting on much more body fat than lean muscle, there is no need to overeat to gain muscle, you just need to be in a calorie surplus at a **moderate** level as I am going to explain in further chapters.

I would suggest changing the phrase to: eat smart to get big. By smart I mean counting the macros of each meal, having enough protein to allow your muscles to recover, having enough carbohydrates to fuel your workouts, the correct amount of fats to maintain healthy testosterone levels and yes, being in a caloric surplus at a moderate level. The key word here is **moderate**, you need around 300, 500 calories over what your body burns each day.

So forget about eating huge amounts of meals and calories to gain muscle, that is simple not true.

3.1.2 Mistake 2: Paying Too Much Attention To Supplements

I see people over and over worrying too much about what supplements to take, they ask me what supplements do I recommend, and I answer with a question: Is your nutrition on point? Are you counting your macronutrients on a daily basis? How many calories did you have so far? And the answer is always the same: No, No and I don't know.

I can't stress this enough, the best supplement out there is real food. Don't even worry about supplements if your diet is off. There is no supplement that is going to give you grater results than **real food**.

People often forget the meaning of the word *supplements*. They exist to supplement and fill in the gaps in your current diet, not to replace food.

Besides, only a very small number of supplements out there are backed up by science, the rest of them are **useless**. Instead of spending tons of money on worthless supplements you should better spend that money in real food.

Bottom line is: don't go crazy with supplements, remember that they exist to fill in the gaps of your daily diet and that only a very small amount of them (I would say 10%) actually work.

3.1.3 Mistake 3: Not Tracking Caloric Intake

Most people out there don't want to track their caloric intake, they just don't want to be bothered with having to count something or worrying whether they can eat one food or another. Here is the truth though, if you want to lose fat or build muscle you have to regulate your food intake, period.

The underlying scientific principle that we are talking about here is **energy balance**, which refers to the amount of energy you burn every day versus the amount you give your body via food. If you want to build muscle you need to be in a positive energy balance, meaning you need to eat more calories than your body burns each day. If you want to lose fat you need to be in a negative energy balance, meaning you need to eat less calories than your body burns each day.

Chances are you already knew this but, the thing is, most people out there know this and still refuse to watch their caloric intake, why? Because counting your daily caloric intake requires work, and most people are not willing to put in the work to do this.

You need to ask yourself how serious you are about this, counting your calories and macros is the fastest way to build muscle or lose fat, and is the only way you can be in full control of what you are doing. I know it can be hard at first but as I said before, with time and practice you will get used to doing it.

Start by tracking only your calories first and once you get used to that move on to count your protein intake, and once you get used to that move on to count your carbohydrates and fats.

Don't worry, I will put some meal plans examples and explain you how you can create a convenient and easy one that adjusts to your schedule in further chapters.

As I said before It isn't about a *"diet"*, It's about creating healthy and sustainable habits that you enjoy. If you don't enjoy the process chances are you will get back to old habits, so don't lie to yourself, every time you incorporate a new habit ask yourself "Is this something I imagine myself doing for 3 months, 6 months, 1 year?" If the answer is no, then adapt yourself to something you can actually stick through.

3.1.4 Mistake 4: Not Getting Enough Rest

A healthy diet and heavy training won't go a long way without something that is simple, but not always easy: a good night's sleep. Lacking in sleep will have a negative impact on your muscle growth and ability to put your best effort at the gym.

Keep in mind that you stimulate growth by training, but it actually happens during recovery time

Sleep recharges the body's energy pool, giving it the necessary endurance to make it through the roughest workouts. It's not only a matter of physical energy, but also of mental energy. Sleeping allows the central nervous system to fully recover.

During sleep, protein synthesis increases, repairing damaged muscle fibers and building new tissue. This process not only replaces the broken-down muscle tissue, but also adds a new layer of lean mass. So in the end, the body repairs itself and wakes up with more muscle volume.

So, how much sleep do we need? According to the National Sleep Foundation people between 18 and 64 years old need from 7 to 9 hours of sleep. Older Adults, 65 +, need from 7 to 8 hours of sleep.

Now that you know how important sleep is when it comes to building muscle make sure you have at least a good 7 hour sleep every day.

Here are some healthy sleep tips from the National Sleep Foundation:

1. Stick to a sleep schedule, even on weekends.
2. Practice a relaxing bedtime ritual.
3. Exercise daily.
4. Evaluate your bedroom to ensure ideal temperature, sound and light.
5. Sleep on a comfortable mattress and pillows.
6. Beware of hidden sleep stealers, like alcohol and caffeine.
7. Turn off electronics before bed.

3.2 The 3 Laws To Follow If You Want To Build Muscle

3.2.1 Law 1: Making Sure Your Macros Are On Point

As we explained before, a huge mistake people often make is to not track their calories and macronutrients. They don't do this because it requires work (at first) , but believe me it's the fastest way to see results, whether you want to gain muscle or lose fat.

Counting your macros and calories take the guess out of the process, it let you be in full control of what you are doing and also reduce the margin for errors, hence you will be putting on lean muscle mass or losing body fat at a quicker rate.

Whether your goal is to gain lean muscle mass or lose fat, as we explained before, it all comes down to energy balance, meaning if you want to build muscle you need to be in a caloric surplus, if you want to lose fat you need to be in a caloric deficit, it's as simple as that. How you make sure you are on a caloric surplus or a caloric deficit? by counting at least your calories, there is no other way around it.

You don't have to keep an exact counting of your calories and macronutrients, an approximation works just fine. What worked for me at first was to get used to keeping track of just the calories, once I felt comfortable with that I started to count my calories plus my protein intake, and finally I added up my carbs and fats to that. Try to do it this way and if you see that you just can't keep track of all your macronutrients, keep at least count of your calories and protein intake which are the most important.

3.2.2 Law 2: Progressive Overload

In simplest terms, in order to get bigger and stronger you need to continually lift more heavy weights and make your muscles work harder than they are used to. If you don't your muscles will not become any stronger or bigger than they currently are.

Here is a simple example of progressive overload; let's say you perform 1 set of the biceps barbell curl for 20 pounds at 8RM (8 repetitions maximum), but as your training progresses 1 set of 20 pounds for 8 repetitions becomes easier and easier and your biceps size have grown since you first started but they have reached a plateau and stopped getting bigger. What has happened is your biceps muscles have adapted to the demands you placed on them but there is no longer a need for them to try to get bigger and stronger because the demands are no longer sufficient enough. Even if you continued performing 1 set of 20 pounds for 8 repetitions for the rest of your life, your strength and muscle size would never improve beyond a certain point. In order for your biceps muscles to get even bigger and stronger than they presently are you need to place even more demands on them.

How do we accomplish progressive overload? By following these simple principles:

1. **Increase Resistance**: Progressively increase the weight you lift as you become stronger and the weight becomes easier. A good indicator of when to increase the resistance is when you are able to perform more than your target repetitions (e.g. your lifting program calls for sets of 10 repetitions but you are able to get 11).

[20]

2. Increase Repetitions For A Given Exercise: Increase the number of repetitions you perform for a given exercise. Push yourself to do 1 or 2 more reps with the aid of a spotter if necessary. If you are able to get those extra reps completely by yourself and it is higher than your target rep range then you know it's time to increase the resistance (weight).

3. Increase Exercise Intensity: Increased effort and intensity for every single set translates into more weight lifted and/or more repetitions performed and thus a more productive workout because your muscles have been pushed beyond what they are used to. The help of a good training partner, or at the very least a trusted spotter, may be crucial for you to achieve this.

4. Increase Sets: Increase the number of sets you perform for a given exercise. Instead of 2 or 3 sets maybe you'll want to increase to 3 or 4 in order to really fatigue the muscle.

5. Increase Frequency: Increase how often you train a certain muscle or muscle group. This technique is most useful for improving lagging or weak muscles or muscle groups. The traditional approach to training a muscle or muscle group only once a week may not be sufficient enough for every individual to make continual gains. Learn to listen to your body and make sure that muscles have had enough time to recuperate between training sessions before increasing frequency.

So, the next time you hit a plateau in your workout try to incorporate one of the above principles.

3.2.3 Law 3: Consistency

It doesn't matter how good your workout or nutrition is if you cannot stick to it. Let's discuss what makes consistency possible.

Both training and nutrition need to be:

1. Realistic
2. Enjoyable
3. Flexible

Realistic

The first thing you need to consider when planning training is your schedule and time frame.

Bodybuilders and powerlifters with a specific competition date need to have a realistic plan based on the time frame they have before their contest. If you have 8 weeks until a meet, or 24 weeks until a bodybuilding show, you have to design your training plan built around this timeframe.

Even for the recreational trainee, if your target is to look good on the beach next summer, you need to start planning now how long you will be gaining and when you need to start your cut, and how your training should fit in with these goals.

If you have decided that the "optimal approach" is training 6 days a week for two hours a day like your favorite bodybuilder, yet you are a father who works 50 hours a week, has a hobby, and tends to have family commitments on the weekends, that may not be realistic.

You have to start with what you can do, before you decide what you should do. Remember that optimal is not necessarily the same thing as realistic. Always think about fitting your training program to what is sustainable and realistic in your life first, before assessing anything else.

Enjoyable

When you have the "realistic" part in check, the next thing to think about is this "enjoyable" part.

So why is enjoyment so important? I guarantee you that if you take a suboptimal plan that you love, you'll put more effort into it than if you take an optimal plan that doesn't get your juices and your passion flowing.

To take a modern example, think of the rise of Crossfit. It's been successful for a reason people are joining Crossfit gyms and making better progress than they ever have done in years. Why would this be? - Because they're enjoying their training more and thus putting in more effort.

Flexible

Flexibility is a requirement of the previous two conditions. It allows you to enjoy your training, and allows it to be realistic.

You are in this game for the long haul and there will be times when you struggle to train as planned. Maybe work gets in the way, or there is a schedule change due to some family commitment - when these things happen it's important to have flexibility to accommodate the changes and keep making progress towards your goals without giving up or program hopping blindly.

3.3 The 4 Worst Mistakes To Avoid If You Want To Lose Fat

3.3.1 Mistake 1: Not Counting Calories

The number one mistake people make when trying to lose fat is not being on a caloric deficit state. There is no other way around it, if you want to lose fat you need to eat less calories in a day than what your body burns, so counting calories becomes a vital part of the process.

This is the principle behind gaining and losing weight:

Fat stores can't be increased without the provision off excess energy, nor can they be reduced without the restriction of energy

It doesn't matter what you eat or when you eat, as long as you stay in a caloric deficit state for a long period of time. In this regard, a calorie is a calorie. I am not saying that you should be eating nothing but junk food to lose weight, however. While it's true that you can lose weight on pretty much any diet, eating the right foods is what we aim for when trying to maintain optimal body composition. If you want to lose fat and not muscle, then a calorie is not just a calorie.

3.3.2 Mistake 2: Doing Tons Of Cardio To Get Shredded

How many overweight people do you see in your gym doing tons of cardio, week after week, to look exactly the same? I sure see a lot. They think that spending hours in the treadmill is going to make them lose weight regardless of their current diet.

Cardio can speed up the process of burning fat, as long as your nutrition is on point, and you are in a caloric deficit state. Most people that spends hours in the treadmill aren't in a caloric deficit, in spite of all the cardio they are doing.

Let's say your daily caloric goal to lose weight is 1600 calories, and for the day you've been eating 2000 calories so far and decided to spend 40 minutes in the treadmill, burning a good 300 calories, that leaves you in a positive energy balance for the day of 100 calories. Although those 40 minutes of cardio helped reduce the caloric intake for the day it was not enough to leave you in a caloric deficit.

Cardio is an excellent tool to use along with proper nutrition, because it can enhance the fat lose and speed up your metabolism. But don't make the mistake to rely only on cardio to lose fat, food intake comes always first.

3.3.3 Mistake 3: Trying To Spot Reduce Fat

This is one of my favorites, the famous: how to reduce belly fat question. I don't know from where does this misconception come from, but people often think they can reduce fat from specific spots by doing exercises in that particular part of the body. This is simply not true.

Fat loss occurs in a whole-body fashion, your body reduces fat stores all over the body. It doesn't matter how many crunches you do to reduce belly fat, you won't have a six pack if you don't reduce your overall fat percentage.

In fact, the exact same opposite may occur, by targeting a specific muscle to reduce the fat around it can make the muscle to grow bigger, and if you are not on a caloric deficit, the layer of fat that surrounds that muscle group will remain the same, so the end result will be a bigger yet blurrier muscle.

Everybody is different, and everybody stores fat in different places at different amounts, and the way you lose fat it is certainly going to be different than mine, as you get leaner you might see more separation on your arms or thighs while other people might see less fat around their waistline, but rest assured that you can lose as much fat as you want in any part of your body, it just might take you a little bit more time see less fat in the areas that you want, but be patient and let your body lean out according to your genetics, eventually you will get there.

3.3.4 Mistake 4: Lifting Too Light

Another misconception about getting shredded is that you should perform higher reps with lighter weight to "tone" the muscle. This misconception is probably the result of thinking that higher reps means more work performed, which can help you burn more calories.

But it's not necessarily the amount of weight that is used, or the number of repetitions that helps burn the most fat, but the intensity of the workout.

There is a study conducted by the Norwegian University of Sport and Physical Education in 2003 that determined that high intensive interval training elevates post-exercise energy expenditure for 4 hours.

Researches also confirms that using heavier loads in your workouts results in a higher metabolic rate post-workout as compared to light weight, hence more calories burn!

Bottom line is, fat lose depends on how much of a caloric deficit you are on a daily basis, higher reps with lighter weights won't help you to speed up the process at all, what can enhance fat lose is high intensive interval training, that has been proven to increase your metabolic rate, helping you to burn more calories.

3.4 The 3 Laws To Follow If You Want To Lose Weight

3.4.1 Law 1: Being in a caloric deficit state

Being in a caloric deficit for a long period of time will result in fat loss, is as simple as that. It all comes down to energy balance, our energy expenditure for the day has to be greater than the energy consumed.

In regard of weight loss, it doesn't matter what you eat as long as you set a calorie intake correctly, if you maintain a moderate calorie deficit by eating a little bit less energy than what you burn every day, you will lose weight.

So, how much of a calorie deficit should you be in? Anywhere from 300 to 500 calories less than your total daily energy expenditure (TDEE). According to a study conducted by the Norwegian School of Sport Sciences, Oslo, Norway [study], weight loss has to happen gradually at a rate of 1.1 - 2.2 pounds (0.5-1 kg/wk) per week. Losing 1.1 pounds is better in terms of preserving lean body mass (LBM) and performance, that's why we don't want to restrict too many calories.

The approach I advise to follow when losing weight is to start with a calorie deficit of 300 - 500 calories, once you hit a plateau you can restrict from 100 - 200 more calories or you can incorporate high intensive interval training (HIIT) to your workout, one of these two.

Bottom line is, you will need to watch your calorie intake to effectively lose weight. You will have to stay disciplined and consistent throughout the process.

If you do it right, you can lose weight without losing muscle and in some cases even while gaining muscle, we'll get back to that in later chapters, for now all you need to know is that the number one rule for losing weight is being in a moderate caloric deficit state for a long period of time.

3.4.2 Law 2: Create a meal plan that adjust to your schedule

It doesn't matter if eating 6 to 8 meals a day increases or not your metabolism if that is something you can't stick to. When incorporating a new habit to your routine always be realistic and ask yourself: Do I see myself doing this for 4 or 6 months? If the answer is no, then you need to adjust things to fit your daily routine.

The goal is to create healthy eating patterns that we can follow for a long period of time. For example if your schedule allows you to eat only 3 meals per day, and no more than that, then create a meal plan that fits your macronutrients in those 3 meals. As long as you are in a caloric deficit it doesn't matter how many meals per day you eat, you will still lose weight. Now, from a bodybuilding perspective is better to at least eat 3 meals per day, which is something I think pretty much anyone can incorporate to their schedule.

At the time of writing this I am on a cutting phase and what works best for me is to eat anywhere from 3 to 5 meals a day. I have breakfast at 9 am, then a pre-workout/lunch at 1 pm, I have my post workout meal at around 5 pm and my last meal of the day is at 8 pm. Again, this is what works for me, and what adjusts best to my schedule, and thanks to that I've been losing weight while preserving as much lean muscle mass as possible for the last 4 months.

Eat as frequently or infrequently as you like, use meal timing as a tool to make your dieting as enjoyable and convenient as possible. This way, you can stick to your diet, which is what matters in the end.

3.4.3 Law 3: Eat the right number of macronutrients

If your goal is to lose weight regardless of muscle loss, then a calorie is just a calorie, you can eat pretty much anything you want and as long as you are in a caloric deficit you will lose weight. But if you want to retain lean muscle mass while losing weight, well that's a whole different story, in that case the macronutrients in that calorie matter a lot.

If you eat less protein than you should, then you'll lose more muscle than you would if you had eaten a proper amount of protein.

If you restrict your carbohydrates too much, you will feel with less energy than usual and your workout is going to suffer.

If you eat too little fat, your testosterone levels will decline.

As you can see, if you want to maintain as much lean muscle mass as possible when losing weight, what you eat matters. How many macronutrients you need depends on your body composition and the phase you are in, cutting phase requires slightly different macros than a bulking phase. In the following chapters, we will explain the concept of macronutrients and how to set them up for a cutting or bulking phase for optimal results.

Counting macronutrients, may sound complicated but it really isn't, it's the simplest and most effective approach to follow when trying to lose weight or gain muscle.

Chapter 4: Macronutrients

There are three basic nutrients known as macronutrients:

1. *Protein:* composed of various amino acids, provides the building blocks for muscle tissue.

2. *Carbohydrate:* fuel for energy, is composed of a variety of less complex or more complex sugar.

3. *Fat:* the nutrients that contains the most densely packed energy stores.

There is another essential nutrient, *water* constitutes 72 percent of muscles and you should be drinking at least 3 liters (0.8 gallons) of water per day.

4.1 Protein

Protein is in charge of building, repairing and maintaining muscle tissue. It is built from building blocks called amino acids. Our bodies make amino acids in two different ways.

First, we've got essential amino acids, those that the body can't manufacture, and thus we must consume in our diets.

Next, we've got nonessential amino acids, those that the body can usually make for itself.

A quick note on how muscle grows and the role of protein in this process

After you workout, your body repairs or replaces damaged muscle fibers through a cellular process where it fuses muscle fibers together to form new muscle protein strands or myofibrils. These repaired myofibrils increase in thickness and number to create muscle hypertrophy (growth).

For muscle breakdown and growth to occur you must force your muscles to adapt by creating stress that is different from the previous threshold your body has already adapted to.

After the workout is completed, the most important part begins which is adequate rest and providing ample fuel to your muscles so they can regenerate and grow. The process of muscle repair highly depends on the amount of protein we consume everyday, it is the only macronutrient that will help you repair muscle tissue.

Best Protein Sources:

- Eggs
- Fish
- Chicken
- Red meat
- Cow's milk
- Chickpeas
- Beans

4.2 Carbohydrate

Carbohydrates are the body's primary and most easily available source of energy. Carbohydrates are essential in our diet for a number of reasons:

1. They are a primary form of energy. The carbohydrates stored in the muscles as glycogen are what allow you to do heavy and intense weight training.

2. Muscle size increased when the body stores glycogen and water in the individual muscle cells.

3. Carbohydrates in the body have a "protein-sparing" effect, keeping the body from burning up excessive protein for energy.

4. The carbohydrate glucose is the main source of energy that fuels the functioning of the brain, and deprivation can have sever effects on mood, personality, and mental ability.

Best carbohydrate sources:

Sweet Potato
Brown Rice
Chickpeas
Bananas
Greek Yogurt

4.3 Fat

Fats are an essential part of our diet and is important for good health. There are different types of fats, with some fats being healthier than others. To help make sure you stay healthy, it is important to eat unsaturated fats in small amounts as part of a balanced diet.

When eaten in large amounts, all fats, including healthy fats, can contribute to weight gain. Fat is higher in energy (kilojoules) than any other nutrient and so eating less fat overall is likely to help with weight loss.

Fats in the body serve three basic functions:

1. They provide the mayor source of stored energy (body fat).

2. They serve to cushion and protect the major organs.

3. They act as an insulator, preserving body heat and protecting against excessive cold.

Best Fat Sources:

Best Fat Sources
Avocados
Olives
Whole eggs
Fatty Fish
Nuts
Chia Seeds
Olive Oil
Peanuts, peanut oil, peanut butter

Chapter 5: Setting Up Your Macronutrients

5.1 Calories

A calorie is a measurement of potential energy in a food, whether it comes from protein, carbohydrate, or fat.

Calories are what determine the overall body's energy balance, if you eat more calories than what your body burns in a day for a long period of time you will gain weight (in the form of fat and/or muscle), if you eat less calories than what your body burns in a day for a long period of time you will lose weight (in the form of fat and/or muscle).

Regardless of the source, 1 gram of protein contains 4 calories, 1 gram of carbohydrate contains 4 calories as well, and 1 gram of fat contains 9 calories.

5.2 Calculating your BMR (Basal Metabolic Rate)

Your BMR is the number of calories your body burns if you were to stay in bed all day. In other words, your body burns a certain amount of calories regardless of your physical activity, this is called your basal metabolic rate. To calculate our BMR we are going to use the Katch McArdle formula:

$$BMR = 370 + (21.6 \times LBM)$$

LBM refers to *lean body mass*, and it's in kilograms for this calculation. Lean body mass refers to the nonfat components of the human body. You calculate your LBM by subtracting your body fat weight from your total body weight, giving you the weight of everything but your body fat. Here is how it works:

$$LBM = (1 - BF\% \text{ expressed as decimal number}) \times total \ body \ weight$$

For example, I am currently 160 pounds at about 10 percent body fat, so my LBM is calculated like this:

$$LBM = (1 - 0.10) \times 160 => LBM = 0.9 \times 160 => LBM = 144$$

There are 2.2 pounds in a kilogram, so here is the formula to calculate the BMR:

$$LBM = 144 / 2.2 = 65$$

$$BMR = 370 + (21.6 \times 65) => BMR = 1774 \ calories \ per \ day$$

Now that we know how many calories our body burns per day if we were to stay in bed all day, we need to multiply this number for a factor, depending on our activity level. That new number is our TDEE, the total daily energy expenditure which is your BMR plus the energy expended during any physical activity.

We multiply our BMR as follows:

1. by 1.2 if you exercise 1 to 3 hours per week.
2. by 1.35 if you exercise 4 to 6 hours per week.
3. by 1.5 if you exercise vigorously for 6 or more hours per week.

The result number will be a fairly accurate measurement of the total energy your body burns every day.

In our example, I workout 4 to 6 hours per week, so:

TDEE = 1774 x 1.35 => TDEE = 2395 calories per day.

Now that we know how many calories our body burns everyday (taking into account our activity level), we need to set up our macronutrients. Let's do that in the next section.

5.3 Setting up your macronutrients to lose fat.

5.3.1 Practical Example

To lose fat we need to be in a caloric deficit state, following the previous example, how much less than 2395 calories per day should we eat?. Well the answer here is between 300 to 500 hundred calories less than our TDEE.

So to lose fat we need to eat between 1895 to 2095 calories a day.

When you first start cutting, you don't want to increase your caloric deficit more than 500 hundred because we want to lose as little muscle as possible in this process, and the higher the caloric deficit is the higher is the possibility of losing more muscle. In every cutting phase (phase in which you lose fat) it's normal to lose a little bit of muscle, but we want to ensure that the muscle loss is minimal. This is why we don't want to increase the caloric deficit more than 500 hundred (at least at first).

Whenever you reach a plateau in this phase, meaning you are not seeing changes in your weight or a decrease in your body fat percentage, you can increase the caloric deficit by 100 hundred calories or increase your cardio.

So now that we know that we need to eat between 1895 to 2095 calories a day let's calculate our macros. Let's say we choose to eat 1895 calories per day, our macronutrients intake should be:

1. *Protein:* **1.1 - 1.3 grams of protein per pound of body weight per day.** That would give us 160 * 1.1 = 176 grams of protein which translates to 704 calories (there are 4 calories per gram of protein).

2. *Fats:* ***15 – 25% of total calories per day.*** In our example 1895 * 0.20 = 379 calories should come from fat sources. Knowing there are 9 calories per gram of fat we should eat 42 grams of fat per day.

3. *Carbohydrates:* **The remaining calories to fulfill daily requirements.** In our example, we know we need to eat 704 calories from protein plus 379 calories from fat that adds up to 1080 calories. 1895 - 1080 = 815 calories should come from carbohydrate sources. This translates to 203 grams of carbs per day.

5.3.2 Recommendations for a cutting phase

Stick to lean sources of protein (fish, chicken, turkey, red meat), this way you will be able to put together a meal plan that works. If your protein sources contain too much fat, you are going to find it hard to stay in a caloric deficit state with proper macronutrients ratios. In later chapters I am going to explain you how you can put together a meal plan that works for you, eating healthy and being on a diet doesn't mean you can't enjoy your meals.

After a week of sticking to your cutting diet, you should assess how it's going. You should measure your progress based on the following:

- your weight (did it go down, up, or stay the same?)
- your clothes (do they feel looser, tighter, or the same?)
- the mirror (do you look fatter, thinner, or the same?)

5.3.3 How Much Weight Should You Lose Per Week?

In previous chapters, we mentioned a study conducted by the Norwegian School of Sport Sciences [study] concluded the optimal amount of weight to lose per week is 0.5 kg (1.1 pounds) if we want to preserve as much lean muscle mass as possible.

5.4 Setting up your macronutrients to gain lean muscle mass.

5.4.1 Practical Example

To gain lean muscle mass we need to be in a caloric surplus, but how many calories above our TDEE should we eat? the same amount we use for fat loss, anywhere from 300 to 500 calories.

The goal of this phase is to put on lean muscle mass with minimal fat gain. It's completely natural to gain some fat along the process but if done correctly we are going to gain more muscle than fat.

Following up with our previous example where our TDEE is 2395 calories per day, in a bulking phase we need to eat anywhere from 2695 to 2895 calories. Let's say we chose to eat 2695 calories per day, our macronutrients intake should be:

1. *Protein:* **0.8 to 1 gram of protein per pound of body weight.** That would give us 160 grams of protein which translates to 640 calories (there are 4 calories per gram of protein)

2. *Fats:* **20 – 30% of total calories per day.** That would give us 2695 * 0.25 = 673 calories from fat sources. Knowing there are 9 calories per 1 gram of fat that leads us with 74 grams of fat per day.

3. *Carbohydrates:* **The remaining calories to fulfill daily requirements.** So far our calories are 673 + 640 = 1313, we

decided to eat 2695 so we have 1382 calories left for carbs. That would be 345 grams of carbs.

That would be the starting point for a 160 pound-guy in a bulking phase.

Remember that while it's true you have to eat more than you normally would to maximize muscle growth, you don't have to be in a huge caloric surplus as some would have you believe.

In this phase, it's completely normal to look kind of "puffy", that because you are going to hold more water than normal, as you will be eating a substantial amount of carbohydrates. This is just part of the process.

5.4.2 Recommendations for a bulking phase

The biggest mistake I see people making in this phase is that they think of bulking as a license to eat whatever they want whenever they want it, and this leads to an increase in the amount of body fat that they will gain. This will slow down your gains because when we are ready to start a cutting phase we will need more time to cut all the excessive fat storage. The amount of muscle gain in relation of the fat gain should be 1:1, meaning if you put on1 pound of muscle it's ok to have put 1 pound of fat as well.

5.4.3 How Much Weight Should You Gain Per Week?

The same principle that we discussed in the cutting phase applies here as well. We want to gain from 1.1 (0.5 kg) to 2.2 pounds (1kg) max per week. Anything out of that range would be too little or too much.

5.5 A Note On Cutting And Bulking Phases

The above numbers for both cutting and bulking are a starting point for you, chances are that you will gain/lose weight in the first two months and then you will stall. When this happens you need to adjust your numbers, decrease or increase your caloric intake by 100 to 200 calories and asses your weight the next week, has it gone up, down or remain the same?

We explained in why your weight is not the most accurate measure for progress tracking, so along with your weight you should also re calculate your body fat percentage and then estimate how much muscle have you put on or how much fat have you lost.

In regard of how many calories you should eat in days you do not train, you should keep them at maintenance level in our example that would be 2395 calories per day.

5.6 Can You Build Muscle And Lose Fat At The Same Time?

The answer here is Yes and No. You may or may not be able to do it, depending on your body composition, training experience, and more.

If you are new to weightlifting or new to proper weightlifting that emphasizes heavy, compound training with the primary goal of getting stronger over time (progressive overload), then you can build muscle and lose fat at the same time.

The people who can't, or who can only gain an amount of muscle so small that it's negligible, are experienced weightlifters who have several years of proper training.

So, how can you build muscle and lose fat simultaneously if you are a newbie to weight-training? The key is to be in a **moderate caloric deficit**.

It's important that you don't put yourself in too large of a deficit, though, because it can lead to muscle loss, energy and mood crashes, and other problems. That's anywhere from 300 to 500 hundred calories from your TDEE (total daily energy expenditure).

While it's possible to lose fat and build muscle at the same time if you are new to weight-lifting, you can expect to put on much less muscle than if you were in a caloric surplus. The fact that it's possible does not mean it is optimal. I suggest to do cutting and bulking phases depending on your body fat percentage rather than trying to gain muscle and lose fat at the same time, regardless if you are a noob or not.

So, don't be fooled by those who claim that you can gain muscle and lose fat at the same time, while it can be done under very special circumstances (if you are a noob or you are on steroids) it's not the optimal approach to building muscle.

5.7 How to know if you need to gain muscle or lose fat first?

Let me answer this question with another question: What Is Your Current Body Fat Percentage? As I mentioned before, the key to doing a "smart" bulk and ending up with something good to show for it in the end is to avoid gaining excess body fat while you build muscle.

Your diet and weight training routine are the key factors in optimizing this muscle fat gain ratio, but there's actually something else in your control that plays a significant role in this area: your current body fat percentage.

The fatter you are and the higher your body fat percentage gets, the worse your calorie partitioning gets and the more likely your body is to start storing excess calories as fat instead of muscle.

Needless to say, the fatter you are when you start to bulk, the fatter you're going to be when you end it. This will lead to a longer cutting phase in the future, increasing the potential for muscle loss. This also means that you're going to spend a nice amount of time during the year unnecessarily looking like crap.

For all these reasons, starting a bulk when you already have a high body fat percentage it's not a very good idea.

The ideal starting point for a bulk phase is when you are at least somewhat lean. So how lean exactly? For men, this typically means 7-10% body fat (or less).

As a rule of thumb if you are anywhere between 6-10% body fat you can start a bulking phase (the leaner you are the best), once you reached 15-17% body fat you should start your cutting phase.

As you can see it all comes down to your current body fat percentage, if you don't know exactly what yours is try to use the methods I described in chapter 1, if that doesn't work for you just look in the mirror and assess yourself. You should be able to tell at least if you are in an already fat state or if you are somewhat lean. If you are in a fat state try cutting first, otherwise try bulking first, is as simple as that.

I made the mistake in the past of starting a bulking phase when I was already in a fat state (18% body fat) and I hated how I looked for months! When you are already fat and put on some muscle without shredding the body fat, your muscles look smooth and bloated, which is not a good thing. Once I started to cut, I realized that I would have to lose weight for at least 5-6 months if I wanted the muscle loss to be minimal. Doing a such long cutting phase can put a lot of unnecessary stress in your life, and that's not the point of doing this, at all.

To sum up, if you are anywhere between 6-10% body fat (lean or somewhat lean) you can start to put on some muscle by being in a caloric surplus, once you reach 15-17% body fat start cutting.

[49]

Chapter 6: Boost Your Gains With Pre And Post Workout Meals

6.1 Eating Before Your Workout

People often overlook the importance of pre-workout nutrition for long-term muscle-building goals. Let's analyze what happens if we were to train on an empty stomach, first our glycogen stores will be rapidly depleted. Once they are fully depleted our body turns to our muscle as its next closest source of available energy.

Another negative consequence of not having a pre-workout meal is that your performance (intensity and strength) will suffer, thus you won't be able to push yourself to the limit, making the progressive overload principle nearly impossible to achieve.

The end result: you're unable to stimulate your muscle fibers to the breaking point at which they'll form new scar tissue and new muscle mass.

6.1.1 Carbohydrate Ingestion Before Your Workout (1-2 hours before workout)

Carbohydrates are stored in our body in the form of glycogen, and it's the main fuel our body use when we need energy. They will help you to push more weight and reps in your workouts, thus indirectly helping you build more muscle over time.

This is why it's so important to eat from 20-40 grams of slow to moderate-digesting carbohydrates 1-2 hours before our workout.

Some recommended low to moderate carbohydrate sources are brown rice, oatmeal, Ezekiel bread, white rice (long grain) and even whole wheat pasta.

It is also beneficial to have a small but sufficient source of fast-digesting carbs to kick-start your workout. For example, besides 20-40 grams of slow digesting carbs 1-2 hours prior to my workout I eat 200 grams of orange juice 15-20 minutes before my workout which has a good 24 grams of fast-digesting carbohydrates.

6.1.2 Protein Ingestion Before Your Workout (1-2 hours before workout)

Of course, no meal is complete without protein. As the building block of new muscle growth, protein - composed of essential and non-essential amino acids - is vital to maintaining a positive nitrogen balance necessary to stimulate maximum protein synthesis.

Obtaining the correct ratio of amino acids is vital to achieving an anabolic state and the best way of achieving this is by consuming complete protein sources such as egg whites, chicken, turkey and even skim milk.

Another option for people on the run is to consume a whey protein shake, which provides a balanced source of quality amino acids necessary to achieve a positive nitrogen balance. As a general rule, consume between 20 to 40 grams of protein in preparation for your training session.

6.1.3 Supplement Ingestion Before Your Workout (30-45 minutes before workout)

A study conducted by the Department of Sports Fitness and Health [study] concluded that ingesting a pre-workout supplement containing caffeine, B-vitamins, amino acids, creatine, and beta-alanine before exercise delays fatigue while improving reaction time and muscular endurance.

When going for a pre-workout supplement try to stay away from proprietary blends. A "proprietary blend" on a dietary supplement's "Supplement Facts" panel is a list of ingredients that are part of a product formula specific to a particular manufacturer. FDA requires manufacturers to list all of the ingredients in a product on its label, along with the amount of each (in terms of weight), unless the ingredients are part of a proprietary blend—then the specific amount of each individual ingredient in the blend does not have to be listed, only the total. So it is important to be aware that the exact amount of each ingredient in a proprietary blend (or blend or delivery system) is unknown. This is especially important when a proprietary blend contains stimulant or stimulant-like ingredients, such as caffeine.

A good pre-workout supplement should have anywhere from 150mg to 300mg (max) of caffeine, 2 to 4 grams of beta alanine, and at least 6 grams of citrulline malate. You should also get anywhere from 3-5 grams of creatine before your workout.

That's it for pre-workout nutrition: 20-40 grams of carbohydrates, 20-40 grams of protein 1-2 hours before workout and a pre-workout supplement 30-45 minutes prior to your workout.

6.2 Eating After Your Workout

The post-workout nutrition is where the majority of bodybuilders place a greater emphasis on.

You probably are aware that if you don't eat protein and/or carbs after training, you'll either impair muscle growth or miss out on the opportunity to accelerate it.

But, why is that post-workout nutrition is so important? Well, when you workout you start a process whereby muscle proteins are broken down. Although this effect is mild when you workout, it rapidly accelerates thereafter.

When muscle breakdown exceeds the body's ability to synthesize new proteins, muscle loss happens. On the other hand, when the body synthesize more protein molecules than it loses, muscle growth occurs.

We need to think of post-workout nutrition as the possibility of minimizing muscle breakdown and maximizing protein synthesis.

6.2.1 Carbohydrate Ingestion After Workout

The main reason to consume carbs post-workout is to replenish the muscle glycogen that you burned during your workout. And the best way to do this it is to consume high-glycemic (fast-digesting) carbs as soon as possible.

Another good reason to eat carbs after training is to spike insulin levels. Post-workout insulin spike decreases the rate of protein breakdown after training. If we manage to decrease the rate of protein breakdown the protein synthesis rate will be greater, thus muscle growth will occur.

By including carbs in our pos-workout meal not only we will quickly raise insulin levels but also keep them elevated for longer periods of time.

To sum up, carbohydrates play a crucial role in post workout nutrition for the following reasons:

• Replenish glycogen
• Decrease protein breakdown
• Increase protein synthesis

Now that we know the importance of carbohydrates in post-workout nutrition, how much should we eat? Well, a good rule of thumb is to eat anywhere from 30-60 grams of fast-digesting carbs. In terms of when to eat the carbs, I recommend immediately after exercise.

6.2.2 Protein Ingestion After Workout

Eating protein after your workout has been proven to stimulate protein synthesis, and we know that the more time our body spends building up proteins instead of breaking them down, the more muscle we gain as a result.

So, How much should we eat? Although there are studies that concluded that 20 grams of post-workout protein stimulates maximum muscle protein synthesis and larger quantities have not shown to offer added benefits, this won't be enough for everyone. Some people will need more to reach the same level of synthesis.

I recommend eating anywhere from 20-30 grams of fast digestive protein such as whey protein immediately after your workout.

6.3 A Note On Pre and Post Workout Meals

Although pre and post workout meals are the most important ones of the day, don't drive yourself crazy with this. We now know that it is important to have a fair amount of protein and carbs both prior and after your workout but the most important factor when building muscle is to eat well-rounded meals throughout your day.

Pre and Post workout meals won't have any effect if your remaining meals for the day are not on point.

Chapter 7: Meal Planning

7.1 Flexible Dieting: If It Fits Your Macros

Flexible dieting is exactly what it sounds like, the art of eating the foods you enjoy the most at any time you want, as long as at the end of the day you hit the numbers you are supposed to. By numbers I mean your macronutrients intake for the day.

Now, don't get me wrong here, this is not a license to eat whatever you want, whenever you want, not at all. The plan here is not eat as much junk food as possible while staying within your numbers. While this could technically "work" for the sole purpose of building muscle or losing fat, you will experience some important micronutrient deficiencies in the process that will get in the way of your performance in the long run. The fact that you could eat junk food and still lose weight or gain muscle doesn't mean you should.

A good rule of thumb here is to get at least 80 % of your daily calories from whole, minimally processed micronutrient dense food. The remaining 20% percent you can spend it in treats and junk food.

The main goal of this type of diet is to eat foods that you enjoy every day. Making a realistic meal plan that you can stick to in the long term, because if you try to restrict yourself too much at first, believe me you won't last long and sooner or later you will slip back to older/bad habits.

Think of it this way, as long as the vast majority of your daily calories come from healthy foods, feel free to include some treats if you want.

The beauty of flexible dieting is that you don't really need to follow a restricted diet plan every day, for instance, every day I wake up and I know that for breakfast I need to get 30 grams of protein 40 grams of carbs and 5-10 grams of fat, one day I would have scrambled eggs with toasts and a nice glass of orange juice, some other days I would have oatmeal with blueberries and greek yogurt with 20 grams of whey protein in it. I could also have 3 McDonalds beagles to fit those macros, but I would also be consuming a whole lot more calories than the previous two options, and I would have to restrict myself much more the rest of the day.

For the 80% of your calories I personally recommend you stick to lean sources of protein, as they are the ones that have the less amount of calories with higher protein quality. You can vary the sources of protein and carbohydrates as much as you want as long as you eat whole nutritious foods and you stay within your macronutrients intake for the day.

For the remaining 20% of your calories you can spend it any way you want it.

7.2 Planning Your Meals To Be Enjoyable And Effective

The goal of this section is to help you create a meal plan that adjusts to your particular schedule and lifestyle. Thanks to the flexibility you will have in both the foods you can eat and when you can eat them, this is easy to do.

Let's recap some of the principles you need to take into account when creating you meal plan:

- **Get 80% of your calories from whole nutritious foods**.
- **Protein**:
  - High-Protein Meat:
  - Steak
  - Ground Beef
  - Pork Chops
  - Chicken Breast
  - Turkey Breast
  - Tuna, Salmon, Tilapia
  - High Protein Dairy And Eggs
  - Whey Protein
  - Cottage Cheese
  - Eggs
  - Milk
  - Greek Yogurt

- High Protein Seeds
- Soybeans
- Lentils
- Broccoli
- Peas
- Asparagus
- **Carbohydrate**:
- Sweet Potato
- Brown Rice
- Oats
- Banana
- Chickpeas
- Nuts
- Pasta
- **Fat**:
- Almonds
- Avocado
- Salmon
- Whole Eggs
- Peanut Butter
- Olive Oil
- Olives
- Parmesan Cheese

• Eat foods you enjoy

• Include a little treat every now and then

• Eat as frequently as you like

• Eat 20-40 grams of slow digestive carbs and 20-40 grams of protein 1 - 2 hours before your workout

• Eat 30-60 grams of carbs and 20-30 grams of high digestive protein after your workout.

I believe every meal plan needs to adjust to the needs and likes of every person, so first make a list of the foods you like eating the most, they should be within the whole nutritious food category. For me this list looks something like this:

Protein sources I like:

• Chicken Breasts
• Fish, Salmon, Tilapia
• Steak
• Chickpeas
• Whey Protein

Carbohydrates sources I like:

• Sweet Potato
• Brown Rice
• Brown Bread
• Oats
• Pasta

Fat sources I like:

- Avocado
- Olives
- Olive Oil
- Fish

Once you have the list of foods you like the most, ask yourself how many meals per day does your schedule and lifestyle allow you to eat. In my case I like to eat 4 to 5 meals per day, let's say I choose 4 meals per day.

I am currently on a cutting phase, at 10% body fat and 150 pounds. My TDEE (total daily energy expenditure) is 2543 calories per day. Being in a cutting phase means I have to eat 300 to 500 less calories than my TDEE, in my case I eat 2200 calories per day. I eat 1.1 gram of protein per pound of body weight, that leaves us with 165 grams of protein per day. The 15% of my calories are coming from fat sources, so 330 calories should be from fat. There are 9 calories per gram of fat so I need to eat 36 grams of fat per day. The rest of my calories are coming from carbohydrate sources. 165 grams of protein per day are 660 calories, plus the 330 calories from fat add up to 990 calories. I need to eat 2200 - 990 = 1300 calories from carbohydrate (there are 4 calories per gram of carb) which is 325 grams of carbs.

Knowing that, what I like to do is to split up those macronutrients in the amount of meals I eat every day. Following our example each meal should consist of 40 grams of protein, 80-90 grams of carbs and 10 grams of fat.

[62]

Next you should establish at what time do you plan to workout, in my case I train every day at 3pm. I like to have two meals before my training and then 2 meals after my training. If you train in the morning for example you should at least have 1 meal (breakfast) as your pre-workout meal.

I have breakfast at 9 am in the morning, then lunch at 1pm, lets plan our breakfast and lunch (pre-workout meal) then.

Once you decided what food you are going to eat for breakfast, in my case I like to eat scrambled eggs with brown bread toast, a glass of orange juice and a cup of coffee, you have to plan how much of those foods are you going to eat to hit your macros for that meal. You should make a table with the list of the food you choose with the following columns; food name, amount, protein, carbs fat, calories. You can find de macronutrients for each food in myFitnessPal app, or entering a question about the nutritional content of a food in google (for example: "How many calories are in a banana?" or "How much protein is in a chicken breast?") and hit search. The answer will show up in a box at the top of the results, with the option to change the serving size for even more accurate information.

This is how my breakfast table looks like:

Food Name	Amount	Protein	Carbs	Fat	Calories
Eggs	1 large egg (50 grams)	6 grams	0 grams	5 grams	75
Brown Bread	2 slices	5 grams	19 grams	0 grams	100
Oats	40 grams	5.2 grams	22 grams	2.2	138
Orange	100 grams	0 grams	12 grams	0 grams	47

Then you just need to play with the amounts to be within your macronutrients intake for that meal. In my case this is how it looks like:

Food Name	Amount	Protein	Carbs	Fat	Calories
Whole Eggs	3 large egg (150 grams)	18 grams	0 grams	15 grams	225
Egg Whites	3 egg whites	9 grams	0 grams	0 grams	60
Brown Bread	3 slices	7.5 grams	28 grams	0 grams	150
Oats	40 grams	5.2 grams	22 grams	2.2	138
Orange	300 grams	0 grams	36 grams	0 grams	141
TOTAL	-	**39.7 grams**	**86 grams**	**17.2 grams**	**714**

Notice that the numbers don't have to be exactly the amount we are supposed to hit for that meal, that's fine, a close approximation will do the work. Now, let's plan our lunch/pre workout meal for the day.

For lunch, I like to stick to lean protein sources such as chicken, fish or red meat. For carbohydrates, I usually have some brown rice, sweet potato or pasta. Now that we know the foods we want to combine let's find out what their macronutrients are.

Food Name	Amount	Protein	Carbs	Fat	Calories
Chicken Breast	100 grams	31 grams	0 grams	3.6 grams	165
Steak	100 grams	25 grams	0 grams	19 grams	271
Tilapia	100 grams	26 grams	0 grams	2.7 grams	129
Brown Rice	100 grams	2.6 grams	23 grams	0.9 grams	111
Sweet Potato	100 grams	1.6 grams	20 grams	0.1 grams	86
Pasta	100 grams	5 grams	25 grams	1.1 grams	131
Olives	100 grams	0.8	6 grams	11 grams	115

Knowing this, we play with the amounts to hit our macronutrients intake for this meal. Take into account that this is my pre-workout meal so I need to eat 20-40 grams of slow digestive carbs and 20-40 grams of protein.

Food Name	Amount	Protein	Carbs	Fat	Calories
Chicken Breast	100 grams	31 grams	0 grams	3.6 grams	165
Brown Rice	200 gram	5.2 grams	46 grams	1.8 grams	222
Sweet Potato	200 grams	3.2 grams	40 grams	0.2 grams	172
Olives	50 grams	0.4 grams	3 grams	5.2 grams	57.5
TOTAL	-	**39.8 grams**	**89 grams**	**10.8 grams**	**616**

So far this is our macronutrients intake for the day:

Food Name	Amount	Protein	Carbs	Fat	Calories
BREAKFAST					
Whole Eggs	3 large egg (150 grams)	18	0	15	225
Egg	3 egg whites	9	0	0	60

Food Name	Amount	Protein	Carbs	Fat	Calories
Whites					
Brown Bread	3 slices	7.5	28	0	150
Oats	40	5.2	22	2.2	138
Orange	300	0	36	0	141
LUNCH					
Chicken Breast	100	31	0	3.6	165
Brown Rice	200	5.2	46	1.8	222
Sweet Potato	200	3.2	40	0.2	172
Olives	50	0.4	3	5.2	57.5
TOTAL	-	**79.5**	**175**	**23**	**1255**

Let's plan our post-workout meal. For convenience, I like to have a high protein high carb shake, but again you can have whatever you want instead.

Foods I like eating post-workout include: blueberries, oats, whey protein, chia seeds, banana etc.

The macronutrients for those foods looks like this:

Food Name	Amount	Protein	Carbs	Fat	Calories
Whey Protein Powder	30 grams	28 grams	10 grams	0 grams	100
Oats	40 grams	5.2 grams	22 grams	2.2	138
Banana	100 grams	1.1 grams	23 grams	0.3 grams	89
Blueberries	100 grams	0.7 grams	14 grams	0.3 grams	57
Chia Seeds	15 grams	2 grams	5 grams	3 grams	78
TOTAL	-	**37 (g)**	**74 (g)**	**5.8 (g)**	**362**

So far, this is what our macronutrient intake for the day looks like:

Food Name	Amount	Protein	Carbs	Fat	Calories
BREAKFAST					
Whole Eggs	3 large egg (150 grams)	18 grams	0 grams	15 grams	225
Egg Whites	3 egg whites	9 grams	0 grams	0 grams	60
Brown Bread	3 slices	7.5 grams	28 grams	0 grams	150
Oats	40 grams	5.2 grams	22 grams	2.2	138
Orange	300 grams	0 grams	36 grams	0 grams	141
LUNCH					
Chicken Breast	100 grams	31 grams	0 grams	3.6 grams	165

Food Name	Amount	Protein	Carbs	Fat	Calories
Brown Rice	200 grams	5.2 grams	46 grams	1.8 grams	222
Sweet Potato	200 grams	3.2 grams	40 grams	0.2 grams	172
Olives	50 grams	0.4 grams	3 grams	5.2 grams	57.5
POST-WORKOUT MEAL					
Whey Protein Powder	30 grams	28 grams	10 grams	0 grams	100
Oats	40 grams	5.2 grams	22 grams	2.2	138
Banana	100 grams	1.1 grams	23 grams	0.3 grams	89
Blueberries	100 grams	0.7 grams	14 grams	0.3 grams	57
Chia Seeds	15 grams	2 grams	5 grams	3 grams	78
TOTAL	-	116.5 (g)	249 (g)	28.8 (g)	1617

Food Name	Amount	Protein	Carbs	Fat	Calories
TARGET	-	165 grams	302 grams	36 grams	2200
REMAINING	-	48.5 grams	53 grams	7.2 grams	583

Knowing this, here is how my dinner looks like:

Food Name	Amount	Protein	Carbs	Fat	Calories
Tilapia	100 grams	26 grams	0 grams	1.7 grams	129
Chickpeas	90 grams	21 grams	32 grams	1.4	210
White Rice	50 grams	3.4 grams	40 grams	0	170
TOTAL	-	50.4 grams	70 grams	3.1 grams	509

Food Name	Amount	Protein	Carbs	Fat	Calories

Food Name	Amount	Protein	Carbs	Fat	Calories
BREAKFAST					
Whole Eggs	3 large egg (150 grams)	18 grams	0 grams	15 grams	225
Egg Whites	3 egg whites	9 grams	0 grams	0 grams	60
Brown Bread	3 slices	7.5 grams	28 grams	0 grams	150
Oats	40 grams	5.2 grams	22 grams	2.2	138
Orange	300 grams	0 grams	36 grams	0 grams	141
LUNCH					
Chicken Breast	100 grams	31 grams	0 grams	3.6 grams	165
Brown Rice	200 grams	5.2 grams	46 grams	1.8 grams	222
Sweet Potato	200 grams	3.2 grams	40 grams	0.2 grams	172

Food Name	Amount	Protein	Carbs	Fat	Calories
Olives	50 grams	0.4 grams	3 grams	5.2 grams	57.5
POST-WORKOUT MEAL					
Whey Protein Powder	30 grams	28 grams	10 grams	0 grams	100
Oats	40 grams	5.2 grams	22 grams	2.2	138
Banana	100 grams	1.1 grams	23 grams	0.3 grams	89
Blueberries	100 grams	0.7 grams	14 grams	0.3 grams	57
Chia Seeds	15 grams	2 grams	5 grams	3 grams	78
DINNER					
Tilapia	100 grams	26 grams	0 grams	1.7 grams	129
Chickpeas	90 grams	21 grams	32 grams	1.4	210

Food Name	Amount	Protein	Carbs	Fat	Calories
White Rice	50 grams	3.4 grams	40 grams	0	170
TOTAL	-	**166.9 grams**	**320 grams**	**32 grams**	**2126**
TARGET	-	**165 grams**	**302 grams**	**36 grams**	**2200**

7.3 Sample Meal Plans

CUTTING PLAN FOR 160 LBS MALE AT 15% BODY FAT TDEE: 2223 - TARGET CALORIES: 1800 PROTEIN: 192 grams - FATS: 30 grams - CARBS: 190 grams				
Food	Calories	Protein	Carbs	Fat
BREAKFAST				
3 slices of brown bread	150	8.7	30	0
2 whole eggs and 2 egg whites	200	20	0	10
40 grams of oats	138	5.2	22	2.2
TOTAL	488	33.9	52	12.2
LUNCH				
120 grams of chickpeas	300	28	44	0
100 grams of chicken breast	160	31	0	3.6
1 banana	90	1.1	22	0
TOTAL	550	60	66	3.6
WORKOUT				

CUTTING PLAN FOR 160 LBS MALE AT 15% BODY FAT TDEE: 2223 - TARGET CALORIES: 1800 PROTEIN: 192 grams - FATS: 30 grams - CARBS: 190 grams				
Food	Calories	Protein	Carbs	Fat
POST-WORKOUT SHAKE				
2 scoops whey protein	140	40	20	0
30 grams of chia seeds	156	5.8	12.4	9.6
TOTAL	296	45.8	32.4	9.6
DINNER				
150 grams of chicken	240	46	0	7.2
55 grams of pasta	190	6	40	0.5
TOTAL	430	52	40	7.7
TOTALS	**1764**	**192.8**	**212.5**	**33.1**
TARGETS	**1800**	**191.7**	**190.4**	**30**

CUTTING PLAN FOR 180 LBS MALE AT 15% BODY FAT TDEE: 2527 - TARGET CALORIES: 2127 PROTEIN: 216 grams - FATS: 35 grams - CARBS: 237 grams				
Food	Calories	Protein	Carbs	Fat
BREAKFAST				
3 slices of brown bread	150	8.7	30	0
2 whole eggs and 2 egg whites	200	20	0	10
80 grams of oats	276	10.4	44	4.4
TOTAL	626	39.1	74	14.4
LUNCH				
140 grams of turkey meat	238	41	0	7
55 grams of pasta	190	6	40	0

CUTTING PLAN FOR 180 LBS MALE AT 15% BODY FAT
TDEE: 2527 - TARGET CALORIES: 2127
PROTEIN: 216 grams - FATS: 35 grams - CARBS: 237 grams

Food	Calories	Protein	Carbs	Fat
TOTAL	518	47	40	7

PRE-WORKOUT MEAL

120 grams of chickpeas	300	28	44	0
100 grams of chicken breast	160	31	0	3.6
TOTAL	460	59	44	3.6

WORKOUT

POST-WORKOUT SHAKE

2 scoops whey protein	140	40	20	0

CUTTING PLAN FOR 180 LBS MALE AT 15% BODY FAT TDEE: 2527 - TARGET CALORIES: 2127 PROTEIN: 216 grams - FATS: 35 grams - CARBS: 237 grams				
Food	**Calories**	**Protein**	**Carbs**	**Fat**
30 grams of chia seeds	156	5.8	12.4	9.6
TOTAL	296	45.8	32.4	9.6
DINNER				
100 grams of tilapia	125	25	0	2.7
200 grams of sweet potato	172	3	40	0.2
TOTAL	297	28	40	2.9
TOTALS	**2197**	**219**	**230**	**37.5**
TARGETS	**2127**	**216**	**237**	**35**

CUTTING PLAN FOR 200 LBS MALE AT 15% BODY FAT
TDEE: 2752 - TARGET CALORIES: 2352
PROTEIN: 240 grams - FATS: 40 grams - CARBS: 260 grams

Food	Calories	Protein	Carbs	Fat
BREAKFAST				
3 slices of brown bread	150	8.7	30	0
3 whole eggs and 2 egg whites	200	20	0	10
80 grams of oats	276	10.4	44	4.4
1 scoop of whey protein	100	20	10	0
TOTAL	726	59.1	84	14.4
LUNCH				
100 grams of salmon	200	20	0	13
200 grams of brown rice	222	5.2	46	2
2 scoop of whey protein	200	40	20	0
TOTAL	622	65.2	66	15
WORKOUT				

CUTTING PLAN FOR 180 LBS MALE AT 15% BODY FAT TDEE: 2527 - TARGET CALORIES: 2127 PROTEIN: 216 grams - FATS: 35 grams - CARBS: 237 grams				
Food	Calories	Protein	Carbs	Fat
POST-WORKOUT SHAKE				
2 scoops whey protein	140	40	20	0
30 grams of chia seeds	156	5.8	12.4	9.6
80 grams of oats	276	10.4	44	4.4
TOTAL	572	56.2	76.4	11
DINNER				
100 grams of chicken breast	165	31	0	3.6
120 grams of chickpeas	300	28	44	0
TOTAL	465	59	44	3.6
TOTALS	2385	239.5	270	44
TARGETS	2352	240	260	40

BULKING PLAN FOR 160 LBS MALE AT 10% BODY FAT
TDEE: 2223 - TARGET CALORIES: 2750 PROTEIN: 160 grams - FATS: 60 grams - CARBS: 390 grams

Food	Calories	Protein	Carbs	Fat
BREAKFAST				
3 slices of brown bread	150	8.7	30	0
2 whole eggs and 2 egg whites	200	20	0	10
80 grams of oats	276	10.4	44	4.4
TOTAL	626	39.1	74	14.4
LUNCH				
110 grams of pasta	400	12	80	0
100 grams of chicken breast	160	31	0	3.6

BULKING PLAN FOR 160 LBS MALE AT 10% BODY FAT
TDEE: 2223 - TARGET CALORIES: 2750
PROTEIN: 160 grams - FATS: 60 grams - CARBS: 390 grams

Food	Calories	Protein	Carbs	Fat
1 banana	90	1.1	22	0
TOTAL	650	44.1	102	3.6

WORKOUT

POST-WORKOUT SHAKE

1 scoop whey protein	100	20	10	0
30 grams of chia seeds	156	5.8	12.4	9.6
80 grams of oats	276	11.6	48	4.4
1 banana	90	1.1	22	0
TOTAL	632	38.5	92.4	14

BULKING PLAN FOR 160 LBS MALE AT 10% BODY FAT
TDEE: 2223 - TARGET CALORIES: 2750
PROTEIN: 160 grams - FATS: 60 grams - CARBS: 390 grams

Food	Calories	Protein	Carbs	Fat
DINNER				
120 (g) of chickpeas	298	28	44	0
50 (g) of white rice	178	3.4	40	0
100 grams of olives	115	0	6	11
Snickers bar (50g)	244	3.5	30	12
TOTAL	835	35	120	23
TOTALS	**2743**	**156.7**	**388**	**55**
TARGETS	**2750**	**160**	**390**	**60**

BULKING PLAN FOR 180 LBS MALE AT 10% BODY FAT
TDEE: 2646 - TARGET CALORIES: 3000
PROTEIN: 180 grams - FATS: 83 grams - CARBS: 382 grams

Food	Calories	Protein	Carbs	Fat
BREAKFAST				
3 slices of brown bread	150	8.7	30	0
3 whole eggs and 2 egg whites	270	27	0	15
80 grams of oats	276	10.4	44	4.4
TOTAL	696	46.1	74	19.4
LUNCH				
100 grams of white rice	358	8	80	0
100 grams of chicken breast	160	31	0	3.6
200 grams of broccoli	70	5.6	14	0.8
1 banana	90	1.1	22	0
TOTAL	578	47.6	116	4.4

BULKING PLAN FOR 160 LBS MALE AT 10% BODY FAT TDEE: 2223 - TARGET CALORIES: 2750 PROTEIN: 160 grams - FATS: 60 grams - CARBS: 390 grams				
Food	Calories	Protein	Carbs	Fat
WORKOUT				
POST-WORKOUT SHAKE				
1 scoop whey protein	100	20	10	0
30 grams of chia seeds	156	5.8	12.4	9.6
80 grams of oats	276	11.6	48	4.4
100 grams of spinach	23	2.9	3.6	0.4
1 banana	90	1.1	22	0
TOTAL	645	41.4	96	14.4
DINNER				
150 grams of low fat steak	540	37.5	0	30
300 grams of sweet potato	258	4.8	60	0.3

BULKING PLAN FOR 160 LBS MALE AT 10% BODY FAT TDEE: 2223 - TARGET CALORIES: 2750 PROTEIN: 160 grams - FATS: 60 grams - CARBS: 390 grams				
Food	**Calories**	**Protein**	**Carbs**	**Fat**
200 grams of broccoli	70	5.6	14	0.8
50 grams of snickers bar	244	3.5	31.5	12
TOTAL	1112	51.4	105.5	41.1
TOTALS	**3031**	**186.5**	**391**	**79.3**
TARGETS	**3000**	**180**	**382**	**83**

BULKING PLAN FOR 200 LBS MALE AT 10% BODY FAT

TDEE: 2885 - TARGET CALORIES: 3300
PROTEIN: 200 grams - FATS: 90 grams - CARBS: 420 grams

Food	Calories	Protein	Carbs	Fat
BREAKFAST				
3 slices of brown bread	150	8.7	30	0
3 whole eggs and 2 egg whites	270	27	0	15
80 grams of oats	276	10.4	44	4.4
TOTAL	696	46.1	74	19.4
LUNCH				
100 grams of white rice	358	8	80	0
100 grams of chicken breast	160	31	0	3.6
200 grams of broccoli	70	5.6	14	0.8
1 banana	90	1.1	22	0
TOTAL	578	47.6	116	4.4
PRE-WORKOUT SHAKE				

BULKING PLAN FOR 200 LBS MALE AT 10% BODY FAT
TDEE: 2885 - TARGET CALORIES: 3300
PROTEIN: 200 grams - FATS: 90 grams - CARBS: 420 grams

Food	Calories	Protein	Carbs	Fat
1 scoop of whey protein	100	20	10	0
40 grams of oats	138	5.2	22	2.2
1 banana	90	1.1	22	0
TOTAL	328	26.3	54	2.2

WORKOUT

POST-WORKOUT SHAKE

1 scoop whey protein	100	20	10	0
30 grams of chia seeds	156	5.8	12.4	9.6
80 grams of oats	276	11.6	48	4.4
100 grams of spinach	23	2.9	3.6	0.4
1 banana	90	1.1	22	0
TOTAL	645	41.4	96	14.4

DINNER

BULKING PLAN FOR 200 LBS MALE AT 10% BODY FAT
TDEE: 2885 - TARGET CALORIES: 3300
PROTEIN: 200 grams - FATS: 90 grams - CARBS: 420 grams

Food	Calories	Protein	Carbs	Fat
150 grams of low fat steak	540	37.5	0	30
300 grams of sweet potato	258	4.8	60	0.3
200 grams of broccoli	70	5.6	14	0.8
50 grams of snickers bar	244	3.5	31.5	12
TOTAL	1112	51.4	105.5	41.1
TOTALS	**3359**	**212.8**	**446**	**81.5**
TARGETS	**3300**	**200**	**440**	**80**

7.4 Cheat Meals

Sometimes it feels great to just let go. To stop controlling everything and just give in to your impulses. When it comes to dieting, this means not counting calories or macros and just eat whatever you want. The goal of this section is to teach how to have cheat meals without ruining your progress on the way.

First let's explain the concept of cheat meal, the goal here is to eat whatever you want for a particular meal (once a week), without going crazy. Chances are that you will exceed your caloric intake for that day, but you should always try to minimize that surplus of calories.

Although there is no single research study that says cheat meals can speed up your metabolism, eating them can help you psychologically. It is difficult for someone to be on a diet 7 days per week without cheating. Notice that the title of this section is cheat meals not cheat days, and by meals I mean having 1 cheat meal per week. Cheating too frequently can prevent you from reaching your goal, or at least it's going to take you longer to reach it. That being said, cheat meals make your diet as a whole more enjoyable and generally improves dietary compliance and thus long-term results.

Now that we know that how we cheat matters, let's analyze what are the biggest mistakes people make when cheating.

7.4.1 Biggest Mistakes People Make When Cheating

Cheating Too Frequently

We know that at least a good 80% of your diet should consist of whole nutritious foods, the remaining 20% you can spend it anywhere you want, as long as you stay within your daily caloric intake. This does not allow much room for cheating, that's why the ideal amount of cheating per is 1 meal per week, more than that will impair your progress in the long term.

Eating Too Much In A Cheat Meal

Many people don't realize how many calories are in the foods they eat in their cheat meals. Although it's ok not knowing exactly the amount of calories of your cheat meal, you should have a good estimation of how many calories you are eating. Remember that we want to minimize the surplus of calories we eat for that day.

Doing Cheat Days Not Meals

Many people think they can afford having an entire cheat day because they were "good" during the week. Think again. Let me put it this way, if you are trying to lose weight, and you are in a caloric deficit of let's say 400 calories per day, you manage to stick to your diet 6 days of the way, that put you in a -2400 calories for that week. In a cheat day you can have a surplus of 2400 calories easily, that's why I don't advise to do cheat days, at least at first when you are learning the basics of nutrition.

7.4.2 How To Enjoy Cheat Meals Without Ruining Your Diet

Here is my rule of thumb when it comes to cheating: cheat once per week and try not to exceed 150% of your current caloric intake for the day.

This allows you to loosen up and enjoy yourself without losing most or all of the week's weight loss progress.

Another good rule to follow is to save up calories if you want to eat a lot, and why not do some extra cardio the day of your cheat meal. What I do the day I know I am having a cheat meal is to save up calories by eating more or less nothing but protein leading up to it. I also like to do some extra cardio in that day. Believe me the combination of saving up calories and doing some extra cardio lets you minimize the surplus of calories and sometimes even staying within your caloric intake for the day.

Bottom Line

Cheating incorrectly is one of the major reasons so many people "inexplicably" can't lose weight "no matter what they do" with their diets.

They simply don't realize that you can basically starve yourself all week and, in one weekend, put yourself right back at square zero.

Cheat correctly, though, and you can have the best of both worlds: the satisfaction of overeating without the penalty of major fat gain.

From Here Is Up To You

Well, we have come to the end of this book, but I hope this is just the beginning of your fitness journey. I truly believe that if you put in practice the main principles laid out here, you will be in your way to a healthier, bigger and shredded you. You will be able to accomplish all of this without having your entire life revolved around the gym and the kitchen. Enjoy life to the fullest while building a better you.

As you will see, you don't need to have great genetics, use steroids, spend hours at the gym or restrict yourself too much with the food to achieve an amazing physique. What you need is consistency, patient and faith in the process.

The main reason I wrote this book is to help you achieve your desire physique, but also to teach you how you can enjoy the process of doing so. Once you learn how to embrace the process everything becomes easier, and you will get there faster believe me.

I am confident that you will achieve whatever goal you set your mind to, and I hope this book helps you in the process of doing so.

Would You Help Me Out?

First, thank you for buying my book. I am confident that if you put in practice what you have just learnt in this book you will achieve whatever goal you set to yourself.

If you enjoyed this book or you found it useful I'd be very grateful if you'd post a short review on Amazon. Your support really does make a difference and I read all the reviews personally so I can get your feedback and make this book even better.

You can leave me a review by visiting the following url:

Review How To Build Muscle And Lose Fat Fast

Thanks again for your support!

Printed in Great Britain
by Amazon